OSTEOPOROSIS DIET COOKBOOK FOR SENIORS.

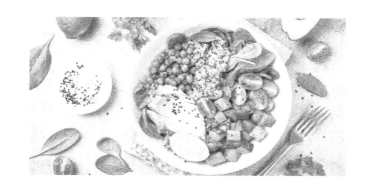

Simple and Savoury Recipes for Stronger Bones and to reverse bone loss naturally.

Oliver Greens.

Copyright @2024 by Oliver Greens.

All rights reserved. No part of this book may be reproduced or transmitted in any form or by any means, electronic or mechanical, including photocopying, recording, or by any information storage and retrieval system, without written permission from the publisher.

CONTENTS

INTRODUCTION . — 5
   CHAPTER ONE: Understanding Osteoporosis. — 9
   What is Osteoporosis? — 9
   Causes of osteoporosis — 10
   Risk Factors of osteoporosis — 11
   Symptoms of osteoporosis — 12
   Diagnosis . — 12
   Treatment. — 13
   Prevention of osteoporosis — 13

CHAPTER TWO: Nutritional Basics For Osteoporosis Management . — 15
   Essential Nutrients For Bone Health — 15
   Recommended Daily Allowance — 21
   Dietary guidelines for seniors with osteoporosis . — 22

CHAPTER THREE: — 26
Foods To Limit For Bone Health. — 26

CHAPTER FOUR:BREAKFAST RECIPES . — 38
   Calcium-Packed Smoothie Bowl. — 38
   Veggie and Cheese Omelette — 42
   Whole Grain Pancakes with Berry Compote — 46
   Yogurt Parfait with Nuts and Seeds — 50

CHAPTER FIVE: Lunch Recipes — 54
   Grilled Salmon Salad — 54
   Quinoa and Vegetable Stir-Fry — 56
   Lentil Soup with Greens — 60
   Chicken and Vegetable Wrap. — 62

CHAPTER SIX:Dinner Recipes. — 66
   Baked Cod with Herbed Quinoa — 66
   Spinach and Mushroom Stuffed Chicken Breast — 69
   Roasted Vegetable and Bean Chili — 74
   Beef and Broccoli Stir-Fry with Brown Rice — 77

CHAPTER SEVEN: SNACKS AND SIDES — 81
   Almond and Date Energy Bites — 81
   Greek Yogurt Dip with Fresh Veggies — 84
   Whole Grain Crackers with Avocado Spread. — 87

CONCLUSION:. — 92
BASIC KITCHEN CONVERSION & EQUIVALENT — 92

INTRODUCTION .

Introducing " Osteoporosis Diet Cookbook for Seniors." This cookbook is designed specifically to empower you, the senior reader, with the knowledge and delicious recipes needed to support your bone health journey. Osteoporosis, a condition characterized by weakening bones, is a significant health concern for many seniors. However, through a well-balanced diet rich in key nutrients, you can take proactive steps to maintain and improve your bone density, ultimately enhancing your overall quality of life.

In this book, we'll explore the critical relationship between diet and osteoporosis, highlighting the key nutrients and dietary strategies that play a pivotal role in supporting bone health. We'll also discuss how this cookbook is structured to help you incorporate osteoporosis-friendly foods into your daily meals effortlessly.

Here is a journey of Kim reserval of Boss Loss through reading a book titled" Osteoporosis Diet Cookbook for Seniors"

As a retired teacher entering her golden years, Kim had always prided herself on her active lifestyle. She enjoyed hiking, gardening, and spending time with her grandchildren. However, when she was diagnosed with osteoporosis, her world turned upside down. Suddenly, every step felt precarious, and the fear of fractures loomed over her like a dark cloud.

Determined to take control of her health, Kim embarked on a quest for knowledge. She devoured books, scoured the internet, and sought advice from healthcare professionals. It was during this search for answers that she stumbled upon a book titled " Osteoporosis Diet Cookbook for Seniors."

Intrigued by the promise of a natural approach to bone health, Mary eagerly delved into the pages of the cookbook. She learned about the critical role that nutrition plays in maintaining strong bones and was inspired by the stories of others who had successfully reversed bone loss through dietary changes.

Armed with newfound knowledge and a collection of osteoporosis-friendly recipes, Kim set out to transform her diet and, in turn, her bone health. She stocked her kitchen with calcium-rich foods like leafy greens, dairy alternatives, and nuts and seeds. She made a conscious effort to incorporate vitamin D-rich foods like fatty fish and fortified dairy products into her meals. And she experimented with new recipes, adding bone-supportive herbs and spices to her favorite dishes.

Over time, Kim began to notice a difference. Her energy levels improved, and she felt more confident in her movements. But the true testament to her progress came during her next bone density scan. To her delight and astonishment, the results showed that her bone density had increased, effectively reversing the bone loss she had experienced.

Kim's journey of transformation serves as a powerful reminder of the impact that simple dietary changes can have on bone health. Through education, determination, and a dash of culinary creativity, she was able to reclaim her strength and vitality, proving that it's never too late to nourish your bones and live life to the fullest.

Key Nutrients for Bone Health

1. Calcium: Essential for bone strength and structure, calcium is a key nutrient in preventing osteoporosis. Dairy products, leafy greens, fortified foods, and certain nuts and seeds are excellent sources of calcium.
2. Vitamin D: Necessary for the absorption of calcium, vitamin D plays a vital role in maintaining bone density. Sunlight exposure, fatty fish, fortified foods, and supplements can help meet your vitamin D needs.
3. Magnesium: Involved in bone formation and density, magnesium supports overall bone health. Green leafy vegetables, nuts, seeds, whole grains, and legumes are excellent sources of magnesium.
4. Protein: Important for maintaining bone strength and preventing muscle loss, protein-rich foods such as lean meats, poultry, fish, eggs, dairy products, legumes, and tofu should be included in your diet.
5. Antioxidants and Anti-inflammatory Compounds: Found in fruits, vegetables, nuts, seeds, and spices, antioxidants and anti-inflammatory compounds help protect bone cells from damage and promote bone health.

About This Cookbook

"Osteoporosis diet cookbook for seniors" is more than just a collection of recipes; it's a comprehensive guide to creating delicious and nutritionally balanced meals that support your bone health goals. Each recipe has been carefully crafted to incorporate osteoporosis-friendly ingredients, ensuring that you receive the essential nutrients your bones need to stay strong and resilient.

Whether you're looking for nutritious breakfast options, satisfying lunch ideas, hearty dinners, or wholesome snacks, this cookbook has you covered. With a diverse range of recipes featuring whole grains, lean proteins, fruits, vegetables, dairy alternatives, and bone-supportive herbs and spices, you'll never have to sacrifice flavor for health.

As you embark on this culinary journey towards better bone health, remember that small changes can make a significant difference. By embracing the principles of this cookbook and making mindful choices about the foods you eat, you can nourish your bones from the inside out and enjoy a vibrant, active lifestyle for years to come.

So, let's dive in and start nourishing our bones together!

CHAPTER ONE: Understanding Osteoporosis.

What is Osteoporosis?

Osteoporosis is a medical condition characterized by weakening of the bones, leading to decreased bone density and increased susceptibility to fractures. In osteoporosis, bone tissue breaks down faster than it can be rebuilt, resulting in bones becoming porous, brittle, and prone to fracture even with minimal trauma. This condition often develops silently over time, without noticeable symptoms until a fracture occurs.

Bone is a living tissue that undergoes constant remodeling, with old bone being removed and replaced by new bone. Osteoporosis disrupts this balance, causing bones to lose density and strength. While osteoporosis can affect any bone in the body, fractures most commonly occur in the hip, spine, and wrist.

Osteoporosis is more common in older adults, particularly women after menopause, due to hormonal changes that affect bone density. However, it can also affect men and younger individuals, especially those with certain medical conditions or lifestyle factors that contribute to bone loss.

Osteoporosis is a significant public health concern worldwide, as fractures resulting from this condition can lead to pain, disability, and reduced quality of life. Prevention, early detection, and appropriate management are essential for reducing the risk of fractures and minimizing the impact of osteoporosis on overall health and well-being. Understanding osteoporosis involves delving into its causes, risk factors, symptoms, diagnosis, treatment, and prevention strategies.

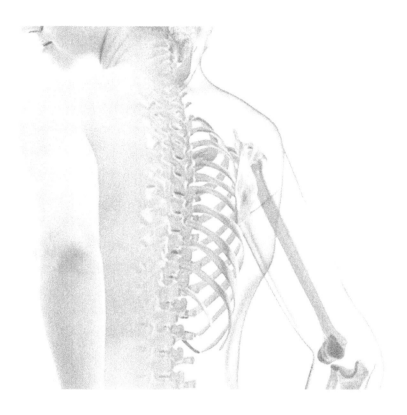

Osteoporosis

Causes of osteoporosis

1. Imbalance in Bone Remodeling: Normal bone is constantly undergoing a process called remodeling, where old bone is removed

and replaced by new bone. Osteoporosis occurs when this process becomes imbalanced, with more bone being resorbed than formed.

2. Hormonal Changes: Hormonal changes, such as those that occur during menopause in women and in individuals with low levels of sex hormones (estrogen in women and testosterone in men), can contribute to bone loss.
3. Nutritional Deficiencies: Inadequate intake of calcium and vitamin D, essential nutrients for bone health, can increase the risk of osteoporosis.
4. Genetic Factors: Family history of osteoporosis or fractures may predispose individuals to the condition.
5. Lifestyle Factors: Sedentary lifestyle, excessive alcohol consumption, smoking, and certain medications (e.g., glucocorticoids) can weaken bones and increase the risk of osteoporosis.

Risk Factors of osteoporosis

- Age: Bone density decreases with age, making older adults more susceptible to osteoporosis.
- Gender: Women, particularly after menopause, have a higher risk of developing osteoporosis due to declining estrogen levels.
- Body Composition: Low body weight or BMI, and a small frame size increase the risk of osteoporosis.
- Medical Conditions: Certain medical conditions like rheumatoid arthritis, hyperthyroidism, and gastrointestinal disorders can predispose individuals to osteoporosis.

- Medications: Long-term use of corticosteroids and some other medications can weaken bones.
- Family History: Having a family history of osteoporosis or fractures increases the likelihood of developing the condition.

Symptoms of osteoporosis

- Fractures: Fragility fractures, particularly in the hip, spine, or wrist, are often the first sign of osteoporosis.
- Loss of Height: Compression fractures in the spine can lead to a stooped posture and a gradual loss of height.
- Back Pain: Pain in the back, caused by collapsed vertebrae or fractures, may occur.

Diagnosis .

- Bone Density Testing: Dual-energy X-ray absorptiometry (DEXA or DXA) scan is the most widely used test to measure bone density and diagnose osteoporosis.
- Medical History and Physical Examination: Evaluating risk factors, symptoms, and medical history aids in diagnosis.

Treatment.

- Medications: Bisphosphonates, hormone therapy (for postmenopausal women), denosumab, and other medications can help slow bone loss and reduce fracture risk.
- Calcium and Vitamin D Supplements: Adequate calcium and vitamin D intake is essential for bone health.
- Lifestyle Modifications: Regular weight-bearing exercise, quitting smoking, limiting alcohol consumption, and maintaining a healthy diet are crucial for managing osteoporosis.
- Fall Prevention: Taking measures to prevent falls can reduce the risk of fractures in individuals with osteoporosis.

Prevention of osteoporosis

- Dietary Changes: Consuming a balanced diet rich in calcium and vitamin D.
- Regular Exercise: Engaging in weight-bearing exercises like walking, jogging, and resistance training helps maintain bone density.
- Healthy Lifestyle: Avoiding smoking and excessive alcohol consumption.
- Bone Density Screening: Regular screening for osteoporosis, especially for individuals at higher risk.

In conclusion, understanding osteoporosis involves recognizing its causes, risk factors, symptoms, diagnosis, treatment, and prevention strategies. By addressing modifiable risk factors and adopting a proactive approach to bone health, individuals can reduce their risk of developing osteoporosis and its associated complications.

CHAPTER TWO: Nutritional Basics For Osteoporosis Management.

Essential Nutrients For Bone Health

Maintaining strong and healthy bones is vital for overall well-being and longevity. Bones provide structure, protect organs, and support muscles, making it crucial to ensure they receive adequate nourishment. Several essential nutrients play key roles in bone health, from building bone density to preventing bone diseases. This comprehensive guide explores these essential nutrients and their significance in maintaining optimal bone health.

1. **Calcium:**
    - Calcium is a primary mineral essential for bone structure and strength.
    - It forms the backbone of bone tissue and contributes to bone density.
    - Adequate calcium intake during childhood and adolescence is crucial for maximizing bone mass. Incorporate these calcium-rich foods into your diet:

    a. Dairy Products:
    - Milk: Opt for low-fat or skim milk for calcium without added saturated fat.

- Yogurt: Choose plain, low-fat yogurt for a calcium-rich snack
- Cheese: Include varieties like mozzarella, cheddar, or cottage cheese for a calcium boost.

  b. Leafy Greens:

  - Kale: Loaded with calcium and other essential nutrients, kale is a versatile addition to salads, soups, and smoothies.
  - Spinach: Add spinach to omelets, pasta dishes, or salads for a nutrient-packed meal.

  c. Fortified Foods:

  - Fortified Plant Milk: Almond, soy, or oat milk fortified with calcium provides a dairy-free alternative.
  - Fortified Cereals: Start your day with fortified breakfast cereals for a calcium-rich morning meal.

2. **Vitamin D:**
   - Vitamin D facilitates calcium absorption and utilization in the body.
   - It helps regulate calcium levels in the blood, promoting bone mineralization.
   - Sunlight exposure triggers vitamin D synthesis in the skin.

- Sources: Fatty fish (salmon, tuna), egg yolks, fortified foods (milk, cereals), sunlight exposure. Vitamin D aids calcium absorption, promoting bone health. Get your daily dose of vitamin D from these sources:

  a. Fatty Fish:
    - Salmon: Rich in vitamin D and omega-3 fatty acids, salmon is an excellent choice for bone health.
    - Mackerel: Incorporate mackerel into your diet for a flavorful source of vitamin D.

  b. Fortified Foods:
    - Fortified Orange Juice: Enjoy a glass of fortified orange juice to boost your vitamin D intake.
    - Fortified Cereals: Look for cereals fortified with vitamin D for an easy way to meet your daily needs.

  c. Sunlight:
    - Spend time outdoors to allow your skin to produce vitamin D naturally. Aim for about 10-15 minutes of sunlight exposure several times a week, taking care to protect your skin from excessive UV radiation.

3. **Vitamin K:**
   - Vitamin K is essential for bone mineralization and formation.

- It helps activate osteocalcin, a protein involved in bone metabolism.
- Adequate vitamin K intake is associated with reduced risk of fractures.
- Sources: Leafy greens (spinach, kale, collard greens), broccoli, Brussels sprouts, fermented foods (natto).:
- Leafy Greens:
  - Swiss Chard: Sauté Swiss chard with garlic and olive oil for a flavorful side dish.
  - Collard Greens: Add collard greens to soups, stews, or stir-fries for a nutritious meal.
- b. Cruciferous Vegetables:
  - Broccoli: Steam or roast broccoli for a vitamin K-rich side dish.
  - Brussels Sprouts: Enjoy roasted Brussels sprouts as a tasty addition to any meal.

4. Magnesium:
- Magnesium supports bone health by assisting in calcium absorption and utilization.
- It contributes to bone density and strength by regulating bone turnover.
- Magnesium deficiency can impair bone quality and increase the risk of osteoporosis.
- Sources: Nuts (almonds, cashews), seeds (pumpkin seeds, sunflower seeds), whole grains, leafy greens, legumes.Magnesium supports bone health by aiding in calcium

absorption and bone formation. Include these magnesium-rich foods in your diet:

a. Nuts and Seeds:

- Almonds: Snack on almonds for a crunchy source of magnesium.
- Pumpkin Seeds: Sprinkle pumpkin seeds on salads or yogurt for a magnesium boost.

b. Whole Grains:

- Brown Rice: Choose brown rice over white rice for a whole grain option rich in magnesium.
- Quinoa: Incorporate quinoa into salads, soups, or stir-fries for a nutritious meal.

c. Dark Chocolate:

- Indulge in dark chocolate with a high cocoa content for a delicious source of magnesium.

5. **Phosphorus:**
   - Phosphorus is a major component of bone mineral hydroxyapatite, providing structural support.
   - It works in conjunction with calcium to maintain bone health.

- Balanced intake of phosphorus is essential for optimal bone mineralization.
- Sources: Dairy products, meat, poultry, fish, nuts, seeds, whole grains.

6. **Vitamin C:**
    - Vitamin C is necessary for collagen synthesis, which forms the matrix of bones.
    - It contributes to bone formation and repair.
    - Adequate vitamin C intake is associated with higher bone mineral density.
    - Sources: Citrus fruits (oranges, lemons), strawberries, kiwi, bell peppers, broccoli.

7. **Vitamin A:**
    - Vitamin A plays a role in bone remodeling and growth.
    - It regulates osteoblast and osteoclast activity, essential for bone turnover.
    - Excessive intake of vitamin A supplements may negatively impact bone health, emphasizing the importance of obtaining it from dietary sources.
    - Sources: Liver, fish oil, dairy products, eggs, orange and yellow fruits and vegetables (carrots, sweet potatoes, pumpkin).

8. **Zinc:**
    - Zinc is involved in bone mineralization and collagen synthesis.
    - It supports bone formation and maintenance.
    - Zinc deficiency can impair bone growth and healing.
    - Sources: Meat, shellfish, legumes, nuts, seeds, dairy products.

Ensuring adequate intake of essential nutrients is vital for promoting optimal bone health throughout life. Calcium, vitamin D, vitamin K, magnesium, phosphorus, vitamin C, vitamin A, and zinc play crucial roles in bone formation, mineralization, and maintenance. A balanced diet rich in these nutrients, along with regular exercise and sunlight exposure, can help prevent bone diseases like osteoporosis and fractures, promoting lifelong skeletal health.

Recommended Daily Allowance

Here are the recommended daily allowances (RDAs) for various essential nutrients related to bone health. The information is presented below in tabular form:

Nutrient	Adults (19-50)	Adults (51+)	Pregnant Women	Breastfeeding Women
Calcium	1000 mg/day	1200 mg/day	1000-1300 mg/day	1000-1300 mg/day
Vitamin D	600 IU/day	800 IU/day	600 IU/day	600 IU/day
Vitamin K	90-120 mcg/day	90-120 mcg/day	No specific RDA	No specific RDA
Phosphorus	700 mg/day	700 mg/day	700 mg/day	700 mg/day
Vitamin C	75-90 mg/day	75-90 mg/day	85 mg/day	120 mg/day

Vitamin A	700-900 mcg RAE/day	700-900 mcg RAE/day	770 mcg RAE/day	1300 mcg RAE/day
Zinc	11 mg/day (men) 8 mg/day (women)	11 mg/day (men) 8 mg/day (women)	11 mg/day	12 mg/day

Please note that the values provided are general recommendations and may vary based on individual factors such as health status, dietary habits, and lifestyle. It's advisable to consult with a healthcare professional or registered dietitian for personalized recommendations.Additionally, obtaining these nutrients from a balanced diet rich in whole foods is generally recommended for optimal health outcomes

- **IU(International Units)**
- **mg(milligrams)**
- **mcg (micrograms)**
- **Retinol Activity Equivalents (RAE)**

Dietary guidelines for seniors with osteoporosis .

Osteoporosis is a common condition characterized by weakened bones, making individuals more susceptible to fractures and other bone-related issues. As seniors are at higher risk of developing osteoporosis due to factors such as aging and hormonal changes, adopting a bone-healthy diet becomes crucial for maintaining skeletal integrity and overall health. Here are guidelines specifically tailored for seniors with osteoporosis, emphasizing nutrient-rich foods and lifestyle strategies to support bone health and well-being.

1. Adequate Calcium Intake:
     - Calcium is essential for building and maintaining strong bones, making it a cornerstone nutrient for individuals with osteoporosis.
     - Seniors with osteoporosis should aim to meet their recommended daily calcium intake through dietary sources such as dairy products (milk, yogurt, cheese), fortified plant-based alternatives, leafy greens (kale, collard greens), tofu, and almonds.
     - Incorporating calcium-rich foods into meals and snacks can help ensure sufficient calcium intake to support bone density and strength.
2. Optimal Vitamin D Levels:
     - Vitamin D plays a crucial role in calcium absorption and utilization, making it essential for bone health.
     - Seniors with osteoporosis should strive to maintain adequate vitamin D levels through a combination of sunlight exposure and dietary sources such as fatty fish (salmon, tuna), egg yolks, fortified foods (milk, cereals), and supplementation if necessary.
     - Regular exposure to sunlight, especially during midday, can help stimulate vitamin D synthesis in the skin, but

supplementation may be required in cases of deficiency or limited sun exposure.

3. Balanced Diet Rich in Nutrients:
   - A well-balanced diet incorporating a variety of nutrient-rich foods is vital for overall health and bone strength.
   - Seniors with osteoporosis should focus on consuming a diet rich in fruits, vegetables, whole grains, lean proteins, and healthy fats to provide essential vitamins, minerals, and antioxidants.
   - Emphasizing foods high in magnesium (nuts, seeds, whole grains, leafy greens), phosphorus (dairy, meat, fish, nuts), vitamin K (leafy greens, broccoli, Brussels sprouts), and vitamin C (citrus fruits, berries, bell peppers) can further support bone health and mineralization.

4. Limiting Sodium and Caffeine:
   - High sodium intake can increase calcium excretion from the body, potentially compromising bone health.
   - Seniors with osteoporosis should aim to reduce their intake of processed and packaged foods high in sodium, opting for fresh, whole foods seasoned with herbs and spices instead.
   - Excessive caffeine consumption may also interfere with calcium absorption and contribute to bone loss, so moderation is key.

5. Regular Physical Activity:
   - Engaging in weight-bearing exercises such as walking, jogging, dancing, and resistance training can help maintain bone density and strength in seniors with osteoporosis.

- Seniors should incorporate regular physical activity into their routine, aiming for at least 150 minutes of moderate-intensity exercise per week, as recommended by health guidelines.

6. Consultation with Healthcare Professionals:
    - Seniors with osteoporosis should work closely with their healthcare providers, including doctors, dietitians, and physical therapists, to develop personalized dietary and lifestyle plans.
    - Regular monitoring of bone health through bone density scans and blood tests can help track progress and inform adjustments to dietary and lifestyle interventions as needed.

CHAPTER THREE:

Foods To Limit For Bone Health.

Maintaining strong and healthy bones is essential for overall well-being, as they provide structural support for the body and protect vital organs. While certain foods contribute positively to bone health, others can have a detrimental effect if consumed excessively or regularly. Here's a detailed overview of foods to limit for bone health:

Sodium-rich Foods:

High sodium intake can lead to calcium loss through urine, which can weaken bones over time. Processed foods, canned soups, salty snacks, and fast food are often loaded with sodium. It's crucial to read food labels and choose low-sodium options whenever possible. Here are some common sodium-rich foods that individuals with osteoporosis may want to moderate or avoid:

- Processed meats: Bacon, sausage, ham, and deli meats often contain high levels of sodium.
- Canned soups and broths: These can be very high in sodium, so it's important to check labels and opt for low-sodium options when possible.
- Processed and packaged foods: Foods like frozen dinners, packaged snacks, chips, and crackers often contain high levels of sodium as a preservative.

- Condiments: Soy sauce, ketchup, barbecue sauce, and salad dressings can be sources of hidden sodium.
- Pickled foods: Pickles, olives, and other pickled vegetables are typically high in sodium.
- Cheese: Some types of cheese, especially processed cheeses and blue cheeses, can contain significant amounts of sodium.
- Baked goods: Commercially baked goods like bread, bagels, and pastries may contain added sodium.

Sodas and Sugary Beverages:

Regular consumption of sugary beverages like sodas, energy drinks, and sweetened fruit juices can adversely affect bone health. These beverages often displace healthier options like water or milk, leading to lower calcium intake. Additionally, excessive sugar consumption can increase the excretion of calcium through urine.

Therefore, individuals with osteoporosis are generally advised to limit or avoid the following types of sugary and soda beverages:

- Regular soda (e.g., cola, lemon-lime soda)
- Fruit-flavored sodas
- Energy drinks with added sugars
- Sweetened iced teas and coffees
- Flavored water with added sugars

- Sports drinks with added sugars

Alcohol:

While moderate alcohol consumption may have some health benefits, excessive alcohol intake can weaken bones and increase the risk of fractures. Alcohol interferes with the body's ability to absorb calcium and disrupts hormonal balance, which is essential for bone health. Limiting alcohol intake is crucial for maintaining strong bones. Here are some types of alcohol that may be of concern:

- Excessive Alcohol Consumption: Heavy alcohol consumption is associated with an increased risk of osteoporosis and fractures. Chronic alcohol abuse can interfere with the body's ability to absorb calcium and other essential nutrients necessary for bone health.
- High-Alcohol Content Beverages: Alcoholic beverages with high alcohol content may contribute to bone loss and increase the risk of fractures. These include:
    - Hard liquors such as whiskey, vodka, rum, gin, and tequila.
    - Spirits with higher alcohol by volume (ABV), as they can have a greater impact on bone health compared to beverages with lower ABV.
- Beer: While moderate consumption of beer may have some health benefits, excessive beer consumption has been linked to decreased bone density. Beer contains compounds called hops, which have

- estrogen-like effects that may affect bone metabolism. Additionally, beer tends to be carbonated, which can potentially interfere with calcium absorption.
- Sweetened Alcoholic Beverages: Cocktails and mixed drinks that contain added sugars or syrups should be consumed in moderation or avoided. These beverages can contribute to weight gain and may have negative effects on overall health, including bone health.
- Caffeinated Alcoholic Beverages: Some alcoholic beverages, such as certain types of cocktails or liqueurs, may contain caffeine. Like caffeine in other forms, excessive consumption of caffeine through alcoholic beverages can increase calcium excretion in the urine, potentially leading to bone loss.
- Wine: While moderate wine consumption has been associated with some health benefits, excessive wine consumption may have negative effects on bone health. Red wine, in particular, contains compounds called polyphenols that may have some protective effects on bone, but excessive intake can negate these benefits

Caffeine:
Found in coffee, tea, energy drinks, and some sodas, caffeine can interfere with calcium absorption and increase calcium excretion in urine when consumed in excess. While moderate caffeine consumption is generally considered safe, individuals with low calcium intake or at risk of osteoporosis should be mindful of their caffeine intake.Here are some

common sources of caffeine that individuals with osteoporosis may want to monitor or avoid:

- Coffee: Coffee is one of the most widely consumed sources of caffeine. Different types of coffee, including espresso, brewed coffee, instant coffee, and specialty coffee drinks, contain varying amounts of caffeine.
- Tea: Tea, including black tea, green tea, white tea, and oolong tea, contains caffeine. The caffeine content in tea can vary based on factors such as the type of tea, brewing time, and water temperature.
- Cola and Other Soft Drinks: Cola beverages, energy drinks, and other soft drinks often contain caffeine. These beverages may also contain added sugars or phosphoric acid, which can potentially have negative effects on bone health.
- Energy Drinks: Energy drinks are popular beverages that often contain high levels of caffeine, along with other stimulants and ingredients. Excessive consumption of energy drinks may have adverse effects on bone health and overall well-being.
- Chocolate and Cocoa Products: Chocolate and cocoa products, including dark chocolate, milk chocolate, and cocoa powder, contain caffeine. The caffeine content in chocolate products can vary depending on factors such as the type of chocolate and the amount consumed.
- Some Medications: Certain over-the-counter and prescription medications, such as some pain relievers, weight loss supplements, and cold medications, may contain caffeine. It's essential to read

medication labels and consult with a healthcare professional if you have concerns about caffeine intake from medications.
- Some Supplements: Some dietary supplements, such as those marketed for energy or weight loss, may contain caffeine or other stimulants. Be cautious when using supplements and check the ingredient list for caffeine content.

High Protein Diets:

Diets excessively high in protein, especially animal protein, may increase calcium excretion and lead to reduced bone density over time. While protein is essential for bone health, particularly for muscle maintenance and repair, it's essential to balance protein intake with adequate calcium and other bone-supporting nutrients.

Consumption of certain types of animal protein may not be ideal for individuals with osteoporosis. Here are some considerations:

- High-Protein Diets: Some high-protein diets, such as those that heavily emphasize animal protein sources while neglecting other essential nutrients like fruits, vegetables, and whole grains, may not be optimal for bone health. These diets often result in increased urinary calcium excretion, potentially leading to a negative calcium balance and bone loss over time.
- Excessive Red Meat Consumption: Red meat, such as beef, lamb, and pork, is a significant source of animal protein. While red meat

contains essential nutrients like iron and zinc, excessive consumption may have negative effects on bone health due to its high sulfur-containing amino acid content. These amino acids can increase the acidity of the blood, leading to calcium loss from the bones to buffer the acidity.

- Processed Meats: Processed meats, including bacon, sausage, hot dogs, and deli meats, are often high in sodium and may contain additives that could potentially affect bone health negatively. Additionally, processed meats have been associated with various health risks, including cardiovascular disease and certain cancers.
- Fried or Grilled Meats: Cooking meat at high temperatures, such as frying or grilling, can lead to the formation of compounds called advanced glycation end products (AGEs), which may have detrimental effects on bone health and overall health. Consuming these types of meats in moderation may be advisable for individuals with osteoporosis.

Highly Acidic Foods:

Foods that promote an acidic environment in the body, such as red meat, processed foods, and refined grains, can potentially leach calcium from bones to help buffer the acidity. While these foods can be part of a balanced diet, it's important to consume them in moderation and pair them with alkaline-forming foods like fruits and vegetables.

Here are some highly acidic foods that individuals with osteoporosis may want to limit or avoid :

- Processed and Packaged Foods: Many processed and packaged foods are highly acidic due to additives and preservatives. These may include:
    - Processed meats (e.g., bacon, sausage, deli meats)
    - Packaged snacks (e.g., chips, crackers, pretzels)
    - Canned soups and sauces
- Soft Drinks and Carbonated Beverages: Soda, cola, and other carbonated beverages are highly acidic due to the presence of carbonic acid. Excessive consumption of these beverages may potentially contribute to bone loss.
- Citrus Fruits: While citrus fruits are rich in vitamin C and other nutrients, they are acidic in nature. Examples include oranges, lemons, limes, grapefruits, and tangerines. While these fruits can be part of a balanced diet, it's advisable to consume them in moderation.
- Tomatoes and Tomato-Based Products: Tomatoes and tomato-based products like tomato sauce and ketchup are acidic. While tomatoes are nutritious and contain lycopene, which may have some benefits for bone health, excessive consumption of acidic tomato products should be avoided.
- Vinegar and Vinegar-Based Foods: Vinegar, including apple cider vinegar and balsamic vinegar, is acidic and may contribute to acidity in the body. Foods pickled or marinated in vinegar should also be consumed in moderation.
- Alcohol: Excessive alcohol consumption can lead to increased acidity in the body. While moderate alcohol consumption may not have a significant impact on bone health for most individuals, excessive intake should be avoided.

- Caffeine: Caffeine-containing beverages like coffee and tea can increase acidity in the body. While moderate consumption is generally considered safe, excessive intake should be avoided, especially if it leads to other health issues.

Excessive Vitamin A:

While vitamin A is essential for vision, immune function, and skin health, excessive intake, primarily from supplements, can negatively impact bone health. High levels of vitamin A have been associated with an increased risk of fractures. It's generally recommended to obtain vitamin A from dietary sources like carrots, sweet potatoes, and leafy greens rather than supplements. Here are some foods that may contain excessive amounts of vitamin A and should be consumed in moderation by individuals with osteoporosis:

- Liver: Liver, particularly beef liver, is one of the richest sources of vitamin A. Consuming large amounts of liver or liver products can lead to excessive vitamin A intake.
- Cod Liver Oil: Cod liver oil is a popular supplement rich in both vitamin A and vitamin D. While vitamin D is important for bone health, excessive intake of vitamin A from cod liver oil may be detrimental to individuals with osteoporosis.
- Fortified Foods: Some processed foods, including breakfast cereals, margarine, and snack bars, may be fortified with vitamin A. While fortification can help address nutrient deficiencies, consuming

excessive amounts of fortified foods may lead to high vitamin A intake.

- Dairy Products: Dairy products like milk, cheese, and yogurt contain small amounts of vitamin A. While these foods are also important sources of calcium and other nutrients beneficial for bone health, excessive consumption may contribute to high vitamin A intake.
- Eggs: Egg yolks contain vitamin A, among other nutrients. While eggs can be part of a balanced diet, individuals with osteoporosis should consume them in moderation to avoid excessive vitamin A intake.
- Some Fish: Certain types of fish, such as salmon, mackerel, and trout, contain vitamin A, particularly in the form of retinol. While fish is a nutritious food choice, excessive consumption of these types of fish may contribute to high vitamin A intake.
- Some Vegetables: Certain vegetables, such as sweet potatoes, carrots, and winter squash, are rich in beta-carotene, a precursor to vitamin A. While beta-carotene is generally considered safe and beneficial for health, consuming very high amounts from these vegetables or supplements may lead to excessive vitamin A levels in the body.

High Oxalate Foods:

Some foods high in oxalates, such as spinach, rhubarb, beet greens, and Swiss chard, can bind to calcium and inhibit its absorption. While these foods offer other nutritional benefits, individuals at risk of kidney stones or with calcium absorption issues may need to moderate their intake.

Here are some high-oxalate foods that individuals with osteoporosis may want to limit or avoid:

- Spinach: Spinach is one of the highest sources of oxalates among leafy greens. While it's nutritious and rich in vitamins and minerals, including calcium, its high oxalate content may make it less ideal for individuals prone to kidney stones or concerned about calcium absorption.
- Beet Greens: Beet greens, the leafy tops of beetroot, are another vegetable high in oxalates. Similar to spinach, they provide various nutrients but may need to be limited for those with concerns about oxalate intake.
- Rhubarb: Rhubarb stalks are high in oxalates. While rhubarb is commonly used in desserts and preserves, individuals with osteoporosis may want to consume it sparingly or avoid it altogether.
- Swiss Chard: Swiss chard is a leafy green vegetable that contains oxalates. While it's a nutritious vegetable, those concerned about oxalate intake may want to moderate their consumption.
- Almonds: Almonds are a healthy snack, but they also contain oxalates. Individuals with concerns about oxalate intake may choose to limit their consumption of almonds and other nuts high in oxalates.
- Chocolate: Cocoa powder and chocolate products contain oxalates. While chocolate is enjoyed by many, individuals with concerns about oxalate intake may want to limit their consumption, particularly if they are prone to kidney stones.
- Tea: Tea, particularly black tea, is another source of oxalates. While tea offers various health benefits, individuals with concerns about oxalate intake may want to moderate their tea consumption.

- Certain Fruits: Some fruits contain moderate levels of oxalates. Examples include figs, berries (such as strawberries, blueberries, and raspberries), and kiwi. While these fruits are nutritious, individuals with concerns about oxalate intake may want to moderate their consumption.

while it's essential to focus on consuming foods that support bone health, such as calcium-rich dairy products, leafy greens, nuts, and seeds, it's equally crucial to limit the intake of foods that can undermine bone strength. By being mindful of these dietary factors and maintaining a balanced diet, individuals can better support their bone health and reduce the risk of osteoporosis.

CHAPTER FOUR: BREAKFAST RECIPES .

Calcium-Packed Smoothie Bowl.

Description:

Indulge in a refreshing and nutritious start to your day with our Calcium-Packed Smoothie Bowl recipe. Bursting with flavor and brimming with essential nutrients, this delightful bowl is a perfect blend of creamy goodness and vibrant freshness.

To craft this invigorating breakfast, begin by gathering your favorite calcium-rich ingredients. Spinach and kale serve as the nutrient-packed base, providing a hearty dose of bone-strengthening calcium. Adding to the green goodness, ripe bananas contribute natural sweetness and a velvety texture, while also delivering potassium for a healthy heart.

For an extra boost of calcium and protein, we incorporate Greek yogurt into the mix. Its creamy consistency not only enhances the smoothie's texture but also provides a satisfyingly rich flavor. To elevate the nutritional profile further, a splash of fortified almond milk lends a subtle nuttiness and an additional calcium kick.

To infuse our smoothie bowl with irresistible flavor, we include a medley of antioxidant-rich berries, such as vibrant strawberries, succulent blueberries, and tart raspberries. These colorful gems not only add sweetness but also bring a burst of freshness and a plethora of vitamins and minerals.

Finally, for a delightful crunch and added nutrition, we sprinkle a handful of calcium-fortified granola atop our smoothie bowl creation. This wholesome addition provides a satisfying texture contrast while contributing additional calcium and fiber.

Garnished with a sprinkle of chia seeds or a drizzle of honey for a touch of sweetness, our Calcium-Packed Smoothie Bowl is a nutritious and delicious way to kick-start your morning routine. Whether enjoyed as a leisurely breakfast at home or as a nourishing on-the-go meal, this vibrant bowl is sure to leave you feeling energized, satisfied, and ready to seize the day ahead

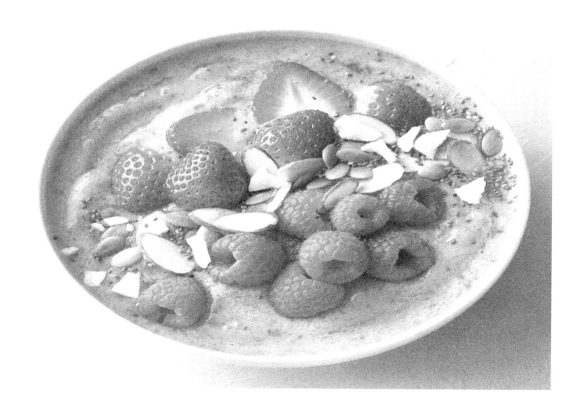

Ingredients .

- 1 cup fresh spinach leaves
- 1 cup kale leaves, stems removed
- 1 ripe banana, sliced
- 1/2 cup Greek yogurt (plain or flavored)
- 1/2 cup fortified almond milk (or any milk of your choice)
- 1/2 cup mixed berries (strawberries, blueberries, raspberries)
- 1/4 cup calcium-fortified granola
- Optional toppings:
    - Chia seeds
    - Honey or maple syrup for drizzling

Instructions:

1. Prepare the Ingredients:
    - Begin by washing the spinach and kale leaves thoroughly under cold running water. Pat them dry with a paper towel or use a salad spinner to remove excess moisture.
    - Slice the ripe banana into small pieces.
    - Rinse the mixed berries under cold water and pat them dry with a paper towel. If using strawberries, hull and slice them.

- Measure out the Greek yogurt, almond milk, and calcium-fortified granola.

2. Blend the Smoothie Base:
    - In a blender, combine the washed spinach leaves, kale leaves (stems removed), sliced banana, Greek yogurt, and fortified almond milk.
    - Blend the ingredients on high speed until smooth and creamy. If the mixture is too thick, you can add more almond milk gradually until you reach your desired consistency.

3. Taste and Adjust:
    - Taste the smoothie base and adjust the sweetness or thickness as desired. If you prefer a sweeter flavor, you can add a drizzle of honey or maple syrup and blend again briefly to incorporate.

4. Prepare the Toppings:
    - Transfer the blended smoothie mixture into a serving bowl.
    - Arrange the mixed berries on top of the smoothie base in an aesthetically pleasing manner.
    - Sprinkle the calcium-fortified granola evenly over the berries to add a delightful crunch and additional calcium boost.

5. Garnish and Serve:
    - Optionally, garnish the smoothie bowl with a sprinkle of chia seeds for added texture and nutritional benefits.
    - If desired, drizzle a small amount of honey or maple syrup over the top for a touch of sweetness and extra flavor enhancement.

6. Serve Immediately:

- Your Calcium-Packed Smoothie Bowl is now ready to be served and enjoyed! Serve it immediately while it's fresh and chilled for the best taste and texture.

7. Optional Customizations:
    - Feel free to customize your smoothie bowl with additional toppings such as sliced fruits (e.g., kiwi, mango, or pineapple), nuts (e.g., almonds, walnuts, or pecans), or seeds (e.g., pumpkin seeds, sunflower seeds) according to your preferences and dietary needs.
8. Clean Up:
    - Rinse out the blender and any other utensils used for preparation with warm soapy water, or place them in the dishwasher for easy cleaning.
    - Enjoy your delicious and nutritious Calcium-Packed Smoothie Bowl, and savor every spoonful of this vibrant and energizing breakfast treat

Veggie and Cheese Omelette

Description:

The veggie and cheese omelet is a delightful combination of fresh vegetables and creamy cheese, folded into fluffy eggs. This versatile dish can be enjoyed for breakfast, brunch, or even a light dinner. Packed with nutrients from various vegetables and protein-rich eggs, it offers a satisfying and wholesome meal option for vegetarians and cheese lovers alike. With its customizable ingredients, you can tailor this omelette to your taste preferences, making it a staple in any kitchen repertoire.

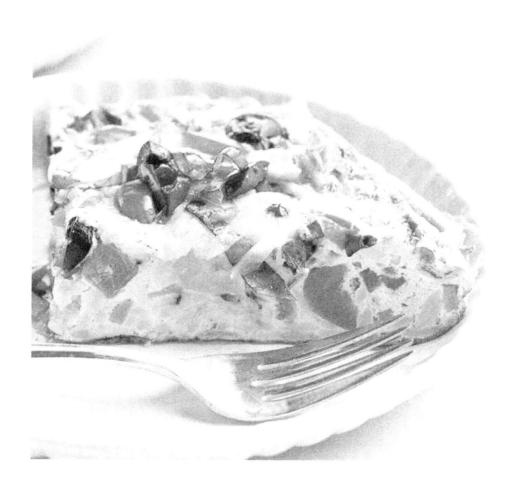

Ingredients:

- 3 large eggs
- 1/4 cup diced bell peppers (red, green, yellow)
- 1/4 cup diced onions
- 1/4 cup sliced mushrooms
- 1/4 cup chopped spinach
- 1/4 cup shredded cheese (cheddar, mozzarella, or your choice)
- Salt and pepper to taste
- 1 tablespoon olive oil or butter for cooking
- Optional: chopped tomatoes, diced zucchini, chopped broccoli, sliced jalapeños, or any other vegetables of your choice

Instructions:

1. Preparation:
   - Wash and chop all the vegetables according to the desired size.
   - Crack the eggs into a mixing bowl and whisk them lightly until well combined. Season with salt and pepper according to taste.
2. Sauté Vegetables:
   - Heat olive oil or butter in a non-stick skillet over medium heat.
   - Add diced onions and sauté until they become translucent, about 2-3 minutes.
   - Add diced bell peppers and sliced mushrooms to the skillet and cook until they are tender, stirring occasionally, for another 3-4 minutes.

- Toss in chopped spinach and any other vegetables you desire, and cook for an additional 1-2 minutes until the spinach wilts and the vegetables are cooked through. Season with salt and pepper to taste.
3. Cooking the Omelette:
    - Once the vegetables are cooked, spread them evenly across the skillet.
    - Pour the whisked eggs over the vegetables, ensuring they cover the entire surface evenly.
    - Allow the eggs to cook undisturbed for a minute or until the edges start to set.
4. Adding Cheese:
    - Sprinkle the shredded cheese evenly over one half of the omelet.
    - Let the omelet continue to cook for another minute or until the cheese begins to melt.
5. Folding and Serving:
    - Using a spatula, gently fold the omelet in half, covering the cheese and creating a half-moon shape.
    - Allow the omelet to cook for an additional 1-2 minutes until the cheese is completely melted and the eggs are cooked to your desired level of doneness.
    - Once cooked, carefully transfer the omelette to a plate.
6. Garnish and Enjoy:
    - Garnish the omelet with additional shredded cheese or fresh herbs if desired.

- Serve hot with toast, a side salad, or your favorite breakfast accompaniments.

Tips:

- Be creative with your vegetable choices to suit your taste preferences or to use up any leftover vegetables in your fridge.
- For a spicier kick, add diced jalapeños or a pinch of red pepper flakes to the vegetable mixture.
- Experiment with different cheese varieties to vary the flavor profile of your omelet.
- Cook the omelet over medium heat to ensure even cooking without burning the eggs or vegetables.

Whole Grain Pancakes with Berry Compote

Description:

Indulge in a wholesome breakfast delight with these Whole Grain Pancakes topped with a vibrant and tangy Berry Compote. These pancakes are not only delicious but also pack a punch of nutrition, thanks to the incorporation of whole grains. Whether you're looking for a nutritious start to your day or a satisfying brunch option, these pancakes are sure to satisfy your cravings and leave you feeling energized.

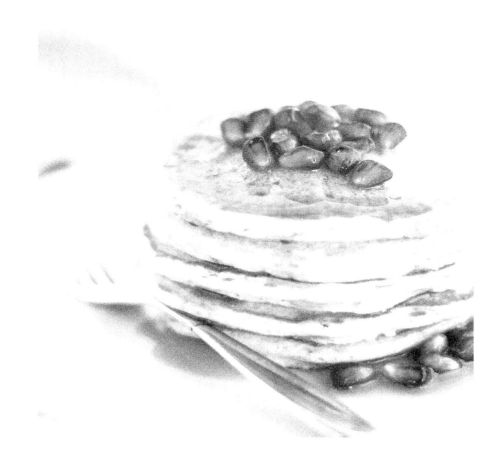

Ingredients:

For Whole Grain Pancakes:

- 1 cup whole wheat flour
- 1/2 cup oat flour
- 2 tablespoons ground flaxseed

- 2 tablespoons honey or maple syrup
- 1 tablespoon baking powder
- 1/4 teaspoon salt
- 1 cup milk (dairy or plant-based)
- 1 large egg
- 2 tablespoons melted butter or oil
- 1 teaspoon vanilla extract

For Berry Compote:

- 2 cups mixed berries (strawberries, blueberries, raspberries, blackberries)
- 2 tablespoons honey or maple syrup
- 1 tablespoon lemon juice
- 1 teaspoon cornstarch (optional, for thickening)

Instructions:

1. Prepare the Berry Compote:

- In a saucepan, combine the mixed berries, honey or maple syrup, and lemon juice.

- Cook over medium heat, stirring occasionally, until the berries begin to break down and release their juices, about 5-7 minutes.
- If you prefer a thicker compote, mix the cornstarch with a tablespoon of water to create a slurry. Stir the slurry into the berry mixture and continue to cook for an additional 2-3 minutes until thickened.
- Remove from heat and set aside while you prepare the pancakes.

2. Make the Whole Grain Pancakes:

- In a large mixing bowl, whisk together the whole wheat flour, oat flour, ground flaxseed, baking powder, and salt.
- In a separate bowl, whisk together the milk, egg, melted butter or oil, honey or maple syrup, and vanilla extract until well combined.
- Pour the wet ingredients into the dry ingredients and stir until just combined. Be careful not to overmix; a few lumps are okay.
- Let the batter rest for 5-10 minutes while you preheat a skillet or griddle over medium heat and lightly grease it with butter or oil.
- Once the skillet is hot, pour about 1/4 cup of batter onto the skillet for each pancake. Cook until bubbles form on the surface of the pancakes and the edges begin to look set, about 2-3 minutes.
- Flip the pancakes and cook for an additional 1-2 minutes on the other side, until golden brown and cooked through.
- Repeat with the remaining batter, greasing the skillet as needed.
- Serve the pancakes warm, topped with the prepared Berry Compote.

3. Serve and Enjoy:

- Plate the Whole Grain Pancakes and generously spoon the warm Berry Compote over the top.
- Optionally, you can add a dollop of Greek yogurt or a sprinkle of chopped nuts for extra texture and flavor.
- Serve immediately and enjoy these nutritious and delicious pancakes with your loved ones.

Yogurt Parfait with Nuts and Seeds

Description:

Elevate your breakfast or snack time with this delightful Yogurt Parfait with Nuts and Seeds. This parfait is a harmonious blend of creamy yogurt, crunchy nuts, and nutritious seeds, creating a satisfying and wholesome treat. Whether enjoyed as a quick morning meal or a satisfying midday snack, this parfait is not only delicious but also packed with protein, fiber, and essential nutrients to fuel your day

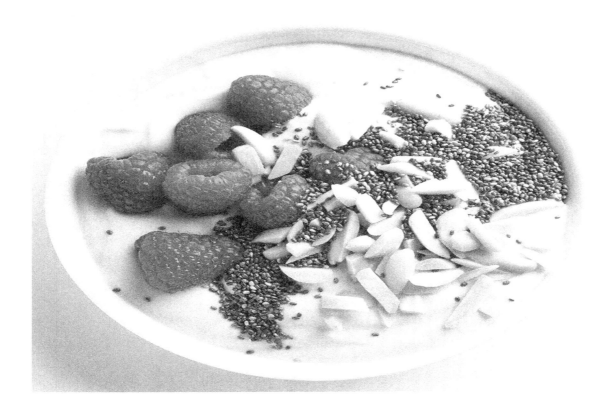

Ingredients:

- 1 cup Greek yogurt (plain or flavored)
- 1/4 cup granola (homemade or store-bought)
- 2 tablespoons chopped nuts (such as almonds, walnuts, or pecans)
- 1 tablespoon mixed seeds (such as chia seeds, flaxseeds, or pumpkin seeds)
- 1 tablespoon honey or maple syrup (optional, for sweetness)

- Fresh fruits (such as berries, sliced bananas, or diced mangoes), optional for layering

Instructions:

1. Prepare the Ingredients:

- If using homemade granola, prepare it in advance according to your preferred recipe and allow it to cool completely.
- Chop the nuts into small pieces if they're not already chopped.
- Measure out the seeds and any other toppings you'd like to include, such as fresh fruits.

2. Assemble the Parfait:

- Start by spooning a layer of Greek yogurt into the bottom of a serving glass or bowl.
- Sprinkle a layer of granola on top of the yogurt.
- Add a layer of chopped nuts and seeds on top of the granola.
- If desired, drizzle a small amount of honey or maple syrup over the nuts and seeds for added sweetness.
- Repeat the layering process until you reach the top of the glass or bowl, alternating between yogurt, granola, nuts, seeds, and any other toppings.
- If using fresh fruits, add a layer of sliced or diced fruits between the other layers or on top of the parfait.

3. Serve and Enjoy:

- Once the parfait is assembled, serve it immediately for optimal freshness and crunchiness.
- Alternatively, you can cover the parfait with plastic wrap and refrigerate it for up to a few hours before serving.
- When ready to serve, garnish the parfait with extra nuts, seeds, or fresh fruits if desired.
- Enjoy this delicious and nutritious Yogurt Parfait with Nuts and Seeds as a satisfying breakfast, snack, or dessert option.

CHAPTER FIVE: Lunch Recipes

Grilled Salmon Salad

Description:

Grilled Salmon Salad is a culinary masterpiece that harmonizes the robust flavor of perfectly grilled salmon with an array of fresh, vibrant ingredients. This dish epitomizes the epitome of healthy indulgence, offering a symphony of textures, colors, and tastes that tantalize the senses. With its delicate balance of protein-rich salmon, crisp greens, and zesty dressing, this salad is not only a feast for the palate but also a celebration of wholesome ingredients.

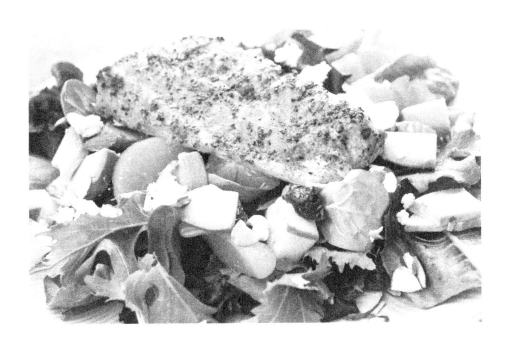

Ingredients:

1. Fresh salmon fillets
2. Mixed salad greens (such as spinach, arugula, and romaine lettuce)
3. Cherry tomatoes
4. Cucumber
5. Red onion
6. Avocado
7. Lemon wedges
8. Olive oil
9. Balsamic vinegar
10. Dijon mustard
11. Honey
12. Salt and pepper
13. Optional additions: toasted nuts (such as almonds or walnuts), crumbled feta cheese, or sliced radishes.

Instructions:

1. Grill the Salmon: Begin by seasoning the salmon fillets with salt, pepper, and a drizzle of olive oil. Preheat the grill to medium-high heat and place the salmon fillets skin-side down. Grill for approximately 4-5 minutes on each side, or until the salmon is cooked through and has a delicious charred exterior. Once done, set aside to cool slightly.

2. Prepare the Salad Greens: Wash and dry the mixed salad greens thoroughly. Tear the larger leaves into bite-sized pieces and place them in a large salad bowl.
3. Chop the Vegetables: Slice the cherry tomatoes in half, thinly slice the cucumber, and finely dice the red onion. Cube the avocado and toss it with a squeeze of lemon juice to prevent browning.
4. Assemble the Salad: Add the grilled salmon, cherry tomatoes, cucumber, red onion, and avocado to the bowl of salad greens.
5. Make the Dressing: In a small bowl, whisk together olive oil, balsamic vinegar, Dijon mustard, honey, salt, and pepper to taste. Adjust the ingredients according to your preference, adding more honey for sweetness or vinegar for tanginess.
6. Toss and Serve: Drizzle the dressing over the salad and gently toss everything together until evenly coated. Be careful not to break up the salmon too much. Garnish with lemon wedges and any optional additions like toasted nuts or crumbled feta cheese if desired.

Quinoa and Vegetable Stir-Fry

Description:

Quinoa and Vegetable Stir-Fry is a delicious and nutritious dish that combines the wholesome goodness of quinoa with a vibrant array of colorful vegetables, creating a flavorful and satisfying meal. This dish is not only packed with essential nutrients but also offers a delightful medley of textures and flavors, making it a favorite among health-conscious individuals and food enthusiasts alike. Whether you're looking for a quick and easy weeknight dinner or a nutritious option for meal prep, this recipe is sure to become a staple in your kitchen.

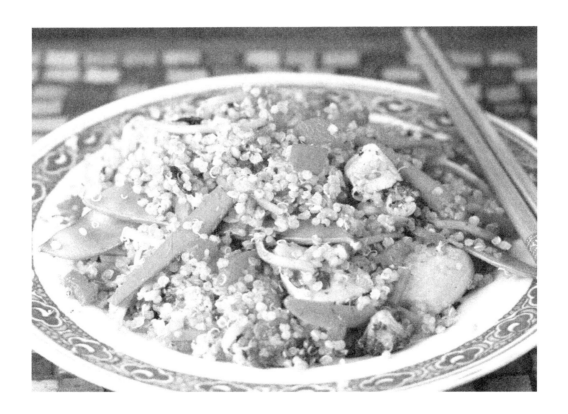

Ingredients:

- 1 cup quinoa, rinsed and drained
- 2 cups water or vegetable broth

- 2 tablespoons olive oil
- 2 cloves garlic, minced
- 1 onion, diced
- 2 carrots, julienned
- 1 red bell pepper, sliced
- 1 yellow bell pepper, sliced
- 1 cup broccoli florets
- 1 cup snap peas, trimmed
- 1 cup sliced mushrooms
- 1 tablespoon soy sauce or tamari (for gluten-free option)
- 1 tablespoon sesame oil
- 2 tablespoons low-sodium soy sauce or tamari (for gluten-free option)
- 1 tablespoon rice vinegar
- 1 teaspoon grated fresh ginger
- Salt and pepper to taste
- Optional garnishes: sliced green onions, sesame seeds, crushed red pepper flakes

Instructions:

1. Cook Quinoa: In a medium saucepan, combine the quinoa and water or vegetable broth. Bring to a boil over medium-high heat, then reduce the heat to low, cover, and simmer for 15-20 minutes, or until the quinoa is cooked and the liquid is absorbed. Remove from heat and let it sit covered for 5 minutes. Fluff with a fork and set aside.

2. **Prepare Vegetables:** While the quinoa is cooking, prepare the vegetables. Heat the olive oil in a large skillet or wok over medium heat. Add the minced garlic and diced onion, and sauté for 2-3 minutes, or until fragrant and translucent.
3. **Add Vegetables:** Add the julienned carrots, sliced bell peppers, broccoli florets, snap peas, and sliced mushrooms to the skillet. Stir-fry for 5-7 minutes, or until the vegetables are tender-crisp.
4. **Make Stir-Fry Sauce:** In a small bowl, whisk together the soy sauce or tamari, sesame oil, low-sodium soy sauce or tamari, rice vinegar, grated ginger, salt, and pepper.
5. **Combine:** Once the vegetables are cooked to your liking, add the cooked quinoa to the skillet, followed by the stir-fry sauce. Stir well to combine, ensuring that the quinoa and vegetables are evenly coated with the sauce. Cook for an additional 2-3 minutes, allowing the flavors to meld together.
6. **Serve:** Remove the skillet from heat. Taste and adjust seasoning if needed. Serve the quinoa and vegetable stir-fry hot, garnished with sliced green onions, sesame seeds, and crushed red pepper flakes if desired.
7. **Enjoy:** Enjoy this nutritious and flavorful dish as a standalone meal or pair it with your favorite protein for added satisfaction. Store any leftovers in an airtight container in the refrigerator for up to 3-4 days.

Lentil Soup with Greens

Description:

Lentil soup with greens is a hearty, nutritious, and comforting dish that combines the earthy flavors of lentils with the vibrant freshness of leafy greens. This soup is not only delicious but also packed with essential nutrients, making it a perfect choice for a wholesome meal. Whether enjoyed as a light lunch or a satisfying dinner, this dish is sure to warm both body and soul, especially on chilly days.

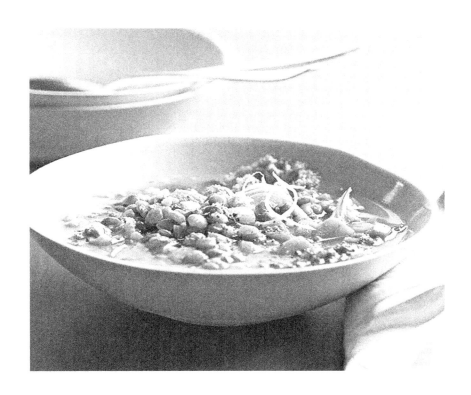

Ingredients:

- 1 cup dried lentils (green or brown), rinsed and drained
- 1 onion, finely chopped
- 2 cloves garlic, minced
- 2 carrots, diced
- 2 celery stalks, diced
- 1 tablespoon olive oil
- 6 cups vegetable broth or water
- 1 bay leaf
- 1 teaspoon dried thyme
- 1 teaspoon ground cumin
- Salt and pepper to taste
- 4 cups leafy greens (such as spinach, kale, or Swiss chard), chopped
- Juice of 1 lemon (optional, for serving)
- Fresh parsley or cilantro, chopped (for garnish)

Instructions:

1. Heat olive oil in a large pot over medium heat. Add chopped onion, garlic, carrots, and celery. Sauté until the vegetables are softened, about 5-7 minutes.
2. Stir in the rinsed lentils, vegetable broth (or water), bay leaf, dried thyme, ground cumin, salt, and pepper. Bring the mixture to a boil.
3. Once boiling, reduce the heat to low and let the soup simmer, partially covered, for about 20-25 minutes or until the lentils are tender.

4. Taste and adjust seasoning if needed. If the soup seems too thick, you can add more broth or water to reach your desired consistency.
5. Stir in the chopped leafy greens (such as spinach, kale, or Swiss chard) and cook for an additional 5 minutes, or until the greens are wilted and tender.
6. Remove the bay leaf from the soup. Squeeze fresh lemon juice over the soup if desired, for a hint of brightness.
7. Ladle the lentil soup into bowls and garnish with fresh chopped parsley or cilantro.
8. Serve hot and enjoy the wholesome goodness of this comforting lentil soup with greens!

Chicken and Vegetable Wrap.

Chicken and vegetable wraps are not only a convenient meal option but also a delicious way to incorporate a variety of flavors and nutrients into your diet. This versatile recipe allows you to customize your wraps according to your preferences, making it suitable for everyone from picky eaters to adventurous foodies. With tender chicken, crunchy vegetables, and a zesty sauce, each bite offers a burst of deliciousness that will leave you craving more. Whether enjoyed at home or on the go, these wraps are sure to satisfy your hunger and tantalize your taste buds.

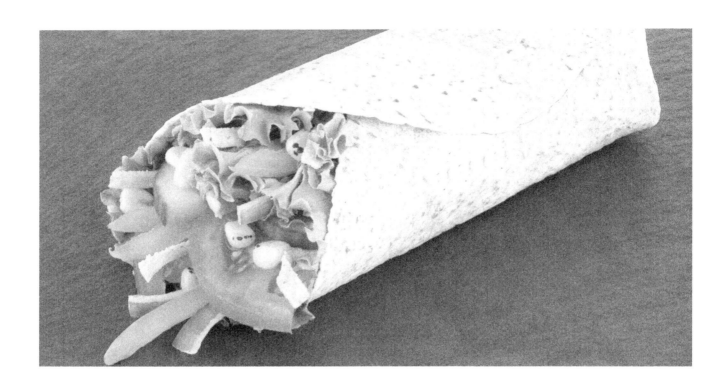

Ingredients:

- 2 boneless, skinless chicken breasts
- 1 tablespoon olive oil
- 1 teaspoon garlic powder
- 1 teaspoon paprika
- Salt and pepper to taste
- 4 large flour tortillas
- 1 cup shredded lettuce
- 1 cup diced tomatoes

- 1/2 cup sliced cucumbers
- 1/2 cup sliced bell peppers (any color)
- 1/4 cup sliced red onions
- 1/2 cup shredded cheese (cheddar, Monterey Jack, or your choice)
- 1/4 cup ranch dressing or your favorite sauce

Instructions:

1. Prepare the Chicken:
    - Slice the chicken breasts into thin strips.
    - In a bowl, mix the olive oil, garlic powder, paprika, salt, and pepper.
    - Add the chicken strips to the bowl and toss until evenly coated with the seasoning mixture.
2. Cook the Chicken:
    - Heat a skillet over medium heat and add the seasoned chicken strips.
    - Cook for 6-8 minutes, or until the chicken is cooked through and no longer pink in the center.
    - Remove the chicken from the skillet and set it aside.
3. Prepare the Wraps:
    - Warm the flour tortillas in the microwave for 10-15 seconds, or until soft and pliable.
    - Lay out each tortilla on a clean surface.
4. Assemble the Wraps:

- Divide the shredded lettuce, diced tomatoes, sliced cucumbers, sliced bell peppers, and sliced red onions evenly among the tortillas.
- Place a portion of the cooked chicken on top of the vegetables on each tortilla.
- Sprinkle shredded cheese over the chicken.

5. Add the Sauce:
   - Drizzle ranch dressing or your favorite sauce over the filling on each tortilla.
6. Wrap the Tortillas:
   - Fold the sides of each tortilla towards the center, then roll it up tightly from the bottom to enclose the filling.
   - Secure each wrap with toothpicks if needed to hold its shape.
7. Serve and Enjoy:
   - Serve the chicken and vegetable wraps immediately, either whole or sliced in half for easier handling.
   - Pair with additional sauce or your favorite side dishes if desired.
   - Enjoy your flavorful and nutritious meal!

CHAPTER SIX: Dinner Recipes.

Baked Cod with Herbed Quinoa

Description:

Baked Cod with Herbed Quinoa is a delightful dish that combines the succulent flavors of flaky cod with the wholesome goodness of quinoa infused with aromatic herbs. This dish offers a perfect balance of protein, healthy fats, and complex carbohydrates, making it both nutritious and delicious. Whether you're cooking for a family dinner or entertaining guests, this recipe is sure to impress with its simplicity and sophisticated flavors.

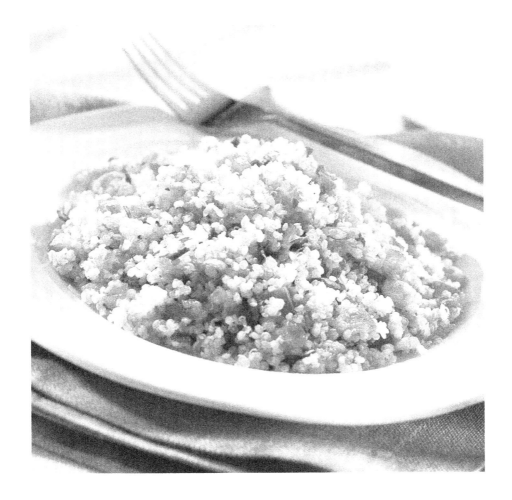

Ingredients:

For the Baked Cod:

- 4 cod fillets (about 6 ounces each), skin removed
- 2 tablespoons olive oil
- 2 cloves garlic, minced
- 1 tablespoon lemon juice
- 1 teaspoon lemon zest
- Salt and pepper to taste
- Fresh parsley, chopped (for garnish)

For the Herbed Quinoa:

- 1 cup quinoa, rinsed
- 2 cups vegetable or chicken broth
- 1 tablespoon olive oil
- 2 cloves garlic, minced
- 1 teaspoon dried thyme
- 1 teaspoon dried rosemary
- 1 teaspoon dried oregano
- Salt and pepper to taste
- Fresh parsley, chopped (for garnish)

Instructions:

1. Preheat the Oven:

   - Preheat your oven to 375°F (190°C).

2. Prepare the Baked Cod:

   - Pat dry the cod fillets with paper towels and place them in a baking dish.
   - In a small bowl, mix together olive oil, minced garlic, lemon juice, lemon zest, salt, and pepper.
   - Drizzle the mixture over the cod fillets, ensuring they are evenly coated.
   - Set aside to marinate while you prepare the herbed quinoa.

3. Prepare the Herbed Quinoa:

   - In a medium saucepan, heat olive oil over medium heat.
   - Add minced garlic and sauté for about 1 minute until fragrant.
   - Stir in the rinsed quinoa and toast it for another 2 minutes.
   - Pour in the vegetable or chicken broth and add dried thyme, rosemary, oregano, salt, and pepper.
   - Bring the mixture to a boil, then reduce the heat to low, cover, and simmer for 15-20 minutes, or until the quinoa is cooked and the liquid is absorbed.

- Once cooked, fluff the quinoa with a fork and adjust seasoning if necessary. Keep warm.

4. Bake the Cod:

- Place the baking dish with the marinated cod fillets in the preheated oven.
- Bake for 12-15 minutes, or until the cod is cooked through and flakes easily with a fork.

5. Serve:

- Once the cod is baked, remove it from the oven.
- Serve the baked cod over a bed of herbed quinoa.
- Garnish with freshly chopped parsley.
- Serve hot and enjoy the delightful flavors of baked cod with herbed quinoa..

Enjoy your Baked Cod with Herbed Quinoa!

Spinach and Mushroom Stuffed Chicken Breast

Description:

Spinach and Mushroom Stuffed Chicken Breast is a delightful dish that combines tender chicken breasts filled with a savory mixture of spinach, mushrooms, and cheese. This flavorful recipe is perfect for a special dinner or a satisfying weeknight meal. The juicy chicken, paired with the earthy flavors of mushrooms and the freshness of spinach, creates a dish that is both elegant and comforting.

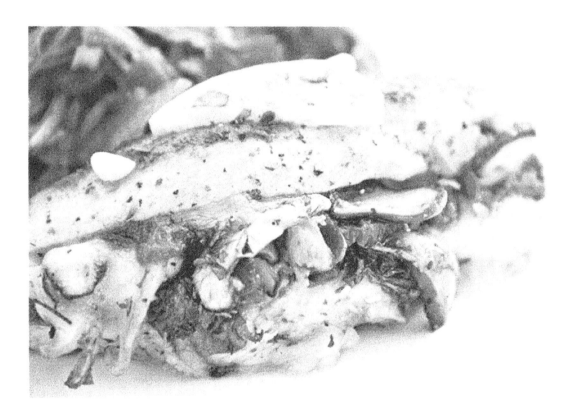

Ingredients:

For the chicken:

- 4 boneless, skinless chicken breasts
- Salt and pepper to taste

- 1 tablespoon olive oil

For the stuffing:

- 2 cups fresh spinach, chopped
- 1 cup mushrooms, finely diced
- 2 cloves garlic, minced
- 1/2 cup ricotta cheese
- 1/4 cup grated Parmesan cheese
- Salt and pepper to taste
- 1/4 teaspoon red pepper flakes (optional)

For the sauce (optional):

- 1 tablespoon butter
- 1 tablespoon all-purpose flour
- 1 cup chicken broth
- Salt and pepper to taste

Instructions:

1. Prepare the chicken breasts:
    - Preheat your oven to 375°F (190°C).

- Place the chicken breasts on a cutting board and use a sharp knife to carefully slice them horizontally, creating a pocket in each breast. Be sure not to cut all the way through.
- Season the chicken breasts with salt and pepper, both inside and out.

2. Make the stuffing:
   - In a skillet, heat the olive oil over medium heat. Add the minced garlic and cook for about 1 minute until fragrant.
   - Add the chopped spinach and mushrooms to the skillet. Cook until the vegetables are softened and any excess liquid has evaporated, about 5-7 minutes.
   - Remove the skillet from the heat and let the mixture cool slightly.
   - Once cooled, transfer the spinach and mushroom mixture to a mixing bowl. Add the ricotta cheese, Parmesan cheese, salt, pepper, and red pepper flakes (if using). Stir until well combined.

3. Stuff the chicken breasts:
   - Divide the spinach and mushroom mixture evenly among the chicken breasts, spooning it into the pockets you created earlier.
   - Secure the openings of the chicken breasts with toothpicks to prevent the stuffing from falling out during cooking.

4. Cook the stuffed chicken breasts:
   - Heat a large oven-safe skillet over medium-high heat. Add a bit of olive oil.

- Carefully place the stuffed chicken breasts in the skillet and cook for 2-3 minutes on each side until they are golden brown.
- Transfer the skillet to the preheated oven and bake for 20-25 minutes, or until the chicken is cooked through and no longer pink in the center.

5. Optional: Make the sauce:
   - While the chicken is baking, you can prepare a simple sauce to serve with it. In a small saucepan, melt the butter over medium heat.
   - Whisk in the flour to create a roux, cooking for 1-2 minutes until golden brown.
   - Gradually whisk in the chicken broth, stirring constantly until the sauce thickens.
   - Season the sauce with salt and pepper to taste.

6. Serve:
   - Once the stuffed chicken breasts are cooked through, remove them from the oven and let them rest for a few minutes.
   - Remove the toothpicks carefully before serving.
   - Optionally, spoon some of the sauce over the chicken breasts before serving.
   - Serve the Spinach and Mushroom Stuffed Chicken Breast hot, garnished with fresh herbs if desired. Enjoy!

Roasted Vegetable and Bean Chili

Description:

Roasted Vegetable and Bean Chili is a hearty and flavorful dish that combines the smoky essence of roasted vegetables with the comforting warmth of chili seasoning. Packed with nutritious ingredients like beans and a variety of vegetables, this chili is both satisfying and wholesome. Whether you're looking for a meatless meal option or simply craving a cozy bowl of chili, this recipe is sure to delight your taste buds and keep you coming back for more.

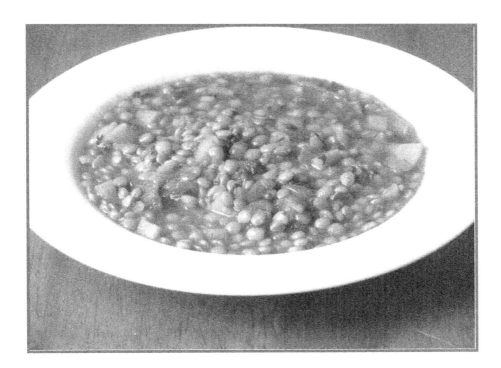

Ingredients:

- 2 cups of mixed beans (such as black beans, kidney beans, and pinto beans), cooked
- 2 bell peppers (red, yellow, or green), chopped
- 1 large onion, diced
- 2 medium carrots, diced
- 2 stalks of celery, diced
- 3 cloves of garlic, minced
- 2 cups of diced tomatoes (fresh or canned)
- 1 can (6 oz) of tomato paste
- 2 tablespoons of chili powder
- 1 tablespoon of smoked paprika
- 1 teaspoon of cumin
- 1 teaspoon of dried oregano
- 1/2 teaspoon of cayenne pepper (adjust to taste)
- Salt and pepper to taste
- 2 tablespoons of olive oil
- 4 cups of vegetable broth
- Fresh cilantro, chopped (for garnish)
- Avocado slices (optional, for garnish)
- Sour cream or Greek yogurt (optional, for garnish)
- Shredded cheese (optional, for garnish)

Instructions:

1. Preheat your oven to 400°F (200°C).
2. In a large bowl, toss the chopped bell peppers, diced onion, diced carrots, diced celery, and minced garlic with olive oil until evenly coated. Spread the vegetables in a single layer on a baking sheet lined with parchment paper.
3. Roast the vegetables in the preheated oven for about 20-25 minutes, or until they are tender and slightly caramelized, stirring halfway through.
4. While the vegetables are roasting, in a large pot or Dutch oven, heat olive oil over medium heat. Add the cooked beans, diced tomatoes, tomato paste, chili powder, smoked paprika, cumin, dried oregano, cayenne pepper, salt, and pepper. Stir well to combine.
5. Pour in the vegetable broth and bring the chili to a simmer. Let it cook for about 15-20 minutes, allowing the flavors to meld together.
6. Once the roasted vegetables are done, add them to the pot with the chili mixture. Stir everything together and let it simmer for an additional 10-15 minutes, allowing the flavors to further develop.
7. Taste and adjust the seasoning if needed, adding more salt, pepper, or spices according to your preference.

8. Serve the roasted vegetable and bean chili hot, garnished with fresh cilantro, avocado slices, sour cream or Greek yogurt, and shredded cheese if desired. Enjoy with crusty bread, rice, or tortilla chips.

Beef and Broccoli Stir-Fry with Brown Rice

Description:

Satisfy your cravings for a wholesome and flavorful meal with this Beef and Broccoli Stir-Fry with Brown Rice. Tender strips of beef, crisp broccoli florets, and savory sauce come together in a symphony of flavors and textures. This dish not only offers a delicious fusion of protein and vegetables but also provides the nutritional benefits of fiber-rich brown rice. Quick to prepare and bursting with Asian-inspired flavors, it's perfect for busy weeknights or weekend dinners.

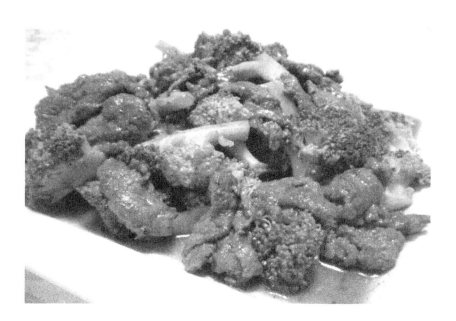

Ingredients:

For the Beef and Broccoli Stir-Fry:

- 1 lb (450g) flank steak, thinly sliced against the grain
- 2 cups broccoli florets
- 3 cloves garlic, minced
- 1 tablespoon fresh ginger, grated
- 2 tablespoons soy sauce (low sodium recommended)
- 1 tablespoon oyster sauce
- 1 tablespoon hoisin sauce
- 1 tablespoon sesame oil
- 2 tablespoons vegetable oil (for cooking)
- Salt and pepper to taste
- Optional: Red pepper flakes for added heat
- Sesame seeds and sliced green onions for garnish

For the Brown Rice:

- 1 cup brown rice
- 2 cups water
- Pinch of salt

Instructions:

1. Prepare the Brown Rice:
   - Rinse the brown rice under cold water until the water runs clear.
   - In a medium saucepan, combine the rinsed rice, water, and a pinch of salt.
   - Bring to a boil over high heat, then reduce the heat to low, cover, and simmer for about 40-45 minutes, or until the rice is tender and the water is absorbed.
   - Once cooked, fluff the rice with a fork and set aside, keeping it warm.
2. Marinate the Beef:
   - In a bowl, combine the thinly sliced flank steak with minced garlic, grated ginger, soy sauce, oyster sauce, hoisin sauce, sesame oil, salt, and pepper. Mix well to ensure the beef is evenly coated.
   - Allow the beef to marinate for at least 15-20 minutes to let the flavors infuse.
3. Stir-Fry the Beef and Broccoli:
   - Heat one tablespoon of vegetable oil in a large skillet or wok over medium-high heat.
   - Once the oil is hot, add the marinated beef slices to the skillet in a single layer. Cook for 2-3 minutes without stirring to allow the beef to sear and brown on one side.
   - Flip the beef slices and add the broccoli florets to the skillet. Cook for an additional 2-3 minutes, stirring occasionally, until

the beef is cooked to your desired doneness and the broccoli is crisp-tender.
    - If desired, sprinkle with red pepper flakes for added heat.
4. Combine and Serve:
    - Once the beef and broccoli are cooked, remove the skillet from the heat.
    - Serve the Beef and Broccoli Stir-Fry hot over a bed of brown rice.
    - Garnish with sesame seeds and sliced green onions for extra flavor and presentation.
    - Enjoy your delicious homemade Beef and Broccoli Stir-Fry with Brown Rice!

CHAPTER SEVEN: SNACKS AND SIDES

Almond and Date Energy Bites

Description.

Almond and Date Energy Bites are delicious and nutritious snacks that provide a quick burst of energy whenever you need it. Packed with wholesome ingredients like almonds, dates, and oats, these bites are not only satisfying but also rich in fiber, protein, and healthy fats. Whether you're fueling up for a workout or simply need a healthy pick-me-up during the day, these energy bites are the perfect solution.

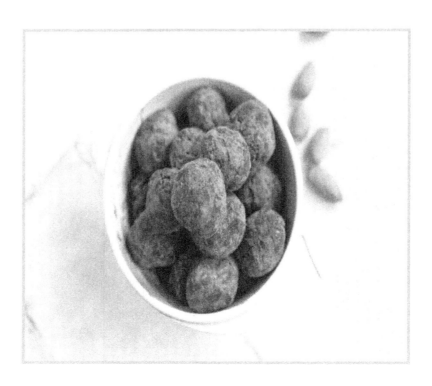

Ingredients.

- 1 cup almonds (raw or roasted)
- 1 cup pitted dates
- 1/2 cup rolled oats
- 2 tablespoons almond butter (or any nut butter of your choice)
- 1 tablespoon honey or maple syrup (optional, for added sweetness)
- 1 teaspoon vanilla extract
- Pinch of salt
- Additional toppings (optional): shredded coconut, cocoa powder, chopped nuts, or dried fruits

Instructions.

1. Prepare the Ingredients:

- If using raw almonds, you can toast them lightly in a dry skillet over medium heat for a few minutes until fragrant. Let them cool before using.
- Make sure the dates are pitted to avoid any pits in the mixture.

2. Combine Almonds and Oats:

- In a food processor or blender, add the almonds and oats. Pulse until they are finely chopped and have a coarse texture. Be careful not to over-process; you want some texture in the bites.

3. Add Dates and Other Ingredients:

- Add the pitted dates, almond butter, honey or maple syrup (if using), vanilla extract, and a pinch of salt to the almond and oat mixture in the food processor.
- Process the mixture until everything is well combined and forms a sticky dough. You may need to scrape down the sides of the processor bowl occasionally to ensure even mixing.

4. Form the Bites:

- Once the mixture has reached a dough-like consistency, it's time to form the energy bites.
- Take about a tablespoon of the mixture and roll it between your palms to form a small ball. If the mixture is too sticky, you can dampen your hands with water to make it easier to handle.
- Continue rolling the mixture into bite-sized balls until all the dough is used up. You should get around 12-15 energy bites, depending on the size.

5. Optional Toppings:

- If desired, roll the energy bites in shredded coconut, cocoa powder, chopped nuts, or dried fruits for extra flavor and texture.

6. Chill and Serve:

- Place the formed energy bites on a baking sheet lined with parchment paper, and refrigerate them for at least 30 minutes to firm up.
- Once chilled, the energy bites are ready to enjoy! Store any leftovers in an airtight container in the refrigerator for up to a week.

7. Enjoy!

- Grab a couple of almond and date energy bites whenever you need a quick and nutritious snack on the go. They're perfect for pre-workout fuel, afternoon pick-me-ups, or satisfying sweet cravings without any guilt

Greek Yogurt Dip with Fresh Veggies

Description.

This Greek Yogurt Dip with Fresh Veggies is a delightful blend of creamy yogurt, savory herbs, and crunchy vegetables. It's the perfect accompaniment to any gathering, whether you're hosting a party or simply craving a healthy snack. Packed with protein and nutrients, this dip offers a refreshing alternative to traditional creamy dips, making it a favorite among health-conscious individuals.

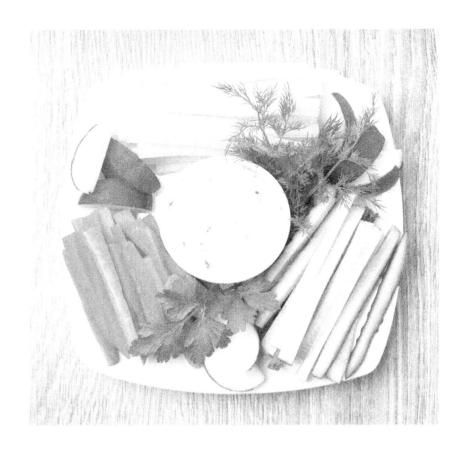

Ingredients.

For the Dip:

- 1 cup Greek yogurt (plain, full-fat or low-fat)
- 1 tablespoon extra virgin olive oil
- 1 clove garlic, minced
- 1 tablespoon fresh lemon juice
- 1 teaspoon lemon zest
- 1 tablespoon fresh dill, finely chopped
- 1 tablespoon fresh parsley, finely chopped

- Salt and pepper to taste

For the Veggie Platter:

- Carrot sticks
- Cucumber slices
- Bell pepper strips (red, yellow, or green)
- Cherry tomatoes
- Celery sticks

Instructions.

1. Prepare the Dip:
   - In a medium-sized mixing bowl, combine the Greek yogurt, extra virgin olive oil, minced garlic, fresh lemon juice, lemon zest, chopped dill, and parsley.
   - Season the mixture with salt and pepper according to your taste preferences.
   - Stir the ingredients until well combined, ensuring that the flavors are evenly distributed throughout the dip.
2. Chill the Dip:
   - Once mixed, cover the bowl with plastic wrap or transfer the dip to an airtight container.
   - Refrigerate the dip for at least 30 minutes to allow the flavors to meld together and enhance the taste.
3. Prepare the Veggie Platter:

- Wash and dry all the vegetables thoroughly.
- Cut the carrots into sticks, slice the cucumber into rounds or sticks, and cut the bell peppers into strips.
- Arrange the prepared vegetables on a serving platter, leaving space in the center for the dip.

4. Serve:
    - Once the dip has chilled and the vegetables are prepared, remove them from the refrigerator.
    - Transfer the Greek yogurt dip to a serving bowl and place it in the center of the vegetable platter.
    - Garnish the dip with a sprig of fresh dill or parsley for an extra touch of freshness.
    - Serve immediately and enjoy the crispness of the vegetables paired with the creamy goodness of the yogurt dip.

5. Storage:
    - If you have any leftover dip, store it in an airtight container in the refrigerator for up to 2-3 days. Make sure to give it a stir before serving again

Whole Grain Crackers with Avocado Spread.

Description.

Whole grain crackers paired with creamy avocado spread make for a delicious and nutritious snack or appetizer. These crackers offer a satisfying crunch while the avocado spread adds a burst of flavor and healthy fats. Whether you're hosting a gathering or looking for a quick snack, this recipe is sure to please your taste buds and provide you with a boost of energy.

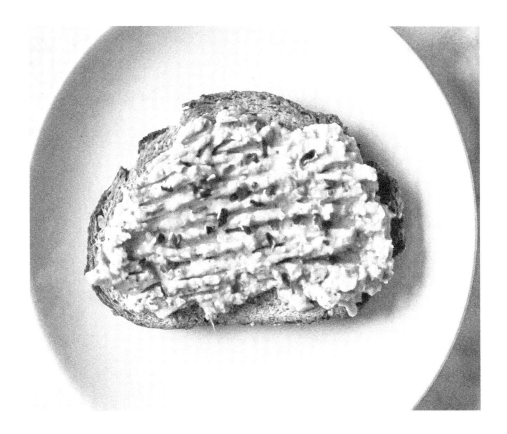

Ingredients.

For the Avocado Spread:

- 2 ripe avocados
- 1 tablespoon fresh lemon juice
- 1 clove garlic, minced

- 1/4 teaspoon salt
- 1/4 teaspoon black pepper
- Optional: pinch of chili flakes for heat

For the Whole Grain Crackers.

- 1 1/2 cups whole grain flour (such as whole wheat or spelt)
- 1/2 teaspoon baking powder
- 1/2 teaspoon salt
- 2 tablespoons olive oil
- 1/2 cup water
- Optional toppings: sesame seeds, poppy seeds, flaxseeds, or sea salt flakes

Instructions.

1. Make the Avocado Spread:

- Cut the avocados in half and remove the pits. Scoop the flesh into a bowl.
- Mash the avocado with a fork until smooth or leave it slightly chunky if you prefer.
- Add lemon juice, minced garlic, salt, black pepper, and chili flakes if using. Mix well to combine.
- Taste and adjust seasoning if needed. Set aside or refrigerate until ready to use.

2. Prepare the Whole Grain Crackers:

- Preheat your oven to 375°F (190°C). Line a baking sheet with parchment paper.
- In a mixing bowl, combine whole grain flour, baking powder, and salt. Stir to combine.
- Add olive oil to the dry ingredients and mix until the mixture resembles coarse crumbs.
- Gradually add water, a little at a time, and mix until a dough forms. You may not need all the water, so add it slowly.
- Knead the dough lightly on a floured surface until smooth.
- Roll out the dough thinly, about 1/8 inch thick. Use a knife or a pizza cutter to cut the dough into squares or rectangles, or use cookie cutters for different shapes.
- Place the crackers on the prepared baking sheet. If desired, sprinkle sesame seeds, poppy seeds, flaxseeds, or sea salt flakes on top of the crackers and gently press them down.
- Bake in the preheated oven for 12-15 minutes or until the crackers are golden brown and crisp.
- Remove from the oven and let cool completely on a wire rack.

3. Assemble and Serve:

- Once the crackers are cooled, spread a generous amount of avocado spread onto each cracker.
- Arrange the avocado-topped crackers on a serving platter.

- Garnish with additional toppings such as freshly ground black pepper or a drizzle of olive oil, if desired.
- Serve immediately and enjoy your delicious whole grain crackers with avocado spread!

Tips.

- Make sure your avocados are ripe for the creamiest spread.
- Experiment with different toppings for the crackers such as dried herbs, grated cheese, or nutritional yeast.
- Store any leftover avocado spread in an airtight container in the refrigerator for up to two days.
- These crackers can be enjoyed on their own or paired with other dips and spreads for a variety of flavor combinations.

Enjoy your wholesome snack of whole grain crackers with creamy avocado spread

CONCLUSION:.

BASIC KITCHEN CONVERSION & EQUIVALENT

DRY MEASUREMENT CONVERSION CHART
- 3 TEASPOONS _1TABLESPOONS_1/16 CUP
- 6 TEASPOONS _ 2 TABLESPOONS _ 1/18 CUP
- 12 TEASPOONS_ 4 TABLESPOONS _ ¼ CUP
- 24 TEASPOONS _ 8 TABLESPOONS _ ½ CUP
- 48 TEASPOONS _ 16 TABLESPOONS _1CUP.

LIQUID MEASUREMENTS CONVERSION CHART.
- 8 FLUID OUNCES _ 1 CUP _ ½ PINT _ ¼ QUART.
- 16 FLUID OUNCES _ 2 CUP _1 PINT _ ½ QUART.
- 32 FLUID OUNCES _ 4 CUP _ 2 PINT _ 1 QUART._1/4 GALLON.
- 128 FLUID OUNCES _16 CUPS _8 PINTS _4QUARTS_1 GALLON.

BUTTER .
- 1 CUP OF BUTTER _2 STICKS _80 OUNCES _239 GRAMS_8 TABLESPOONS.

OVEN TEMPERATURES
- 120°C _ 250F
- 160°C_ 320F

- 180°C _ 350F
- 205°C _ 400F
- 220°C _ 425F

BAKING IN GRAMS.
- 1 CUP OF FLOUR _140 GRAMS
- 1 CUP OF SUGAR _ 150 GRAMS
- 1 CUP OF POWDERED SUGAR _ 160 GRAMS

VOLUME .
- 1 MILLIMETRE_ ⅕ TEASPOON
- 5 MILLiMETRES_1 TEASPOON
- 15 MILLIMETRES _1 TABLESPOON
- 240 MILLIMETRES _1 CUP OR 8 FLUID OUNCES

WEIGHT .
- 1 GRAM _.035 OUNCES
- 1 GRAM _ 1.1 POUND
- 1 KILOGRAM_35 OUNCES

METRIC FOR COOKING CONVERSATIONS
- ⅕ **TSP**_ 1ml
- 1 TSP _5ml
- 1 TBSP_15 ml
- 1 FL OUNCE _30 ml
- 1 CUP _ 237 ml

- 1 PINT(2 CUPS)_ 473 ml
- 1 QUART(4 CUPS)_ •95 litre
- 1 GALLON (16 CUPS)_ 3.8 litres
- 1 OZ_ 28 GRAMS
- 1 POUND _454 GRAMS

1 CUP CONVERSIONS

- 1 CUP_ 8 FLUID OUNCES
- 1 CUP _ 16 TABLESPOONS
- I CUP_ 48 TEASPOONS
- 1 CUP _ ½ PINT
- 1 CUP_ ¼ QUART
- 1 CUP _ 1/16 GALLON
- 1 CUP OF VEGETABLE OIL _ 7.7 OZ
- 1 CUP OF ALL_ PURPOSE FLOUR _ 4.5 OZ
- 1 CUP OF BUTTER _8 OZ
- 1 CUP OF MILK _ 8 OZ
- 1 CUP OF HEAVY CREAM _ 8.40 OZ
- 1 CUP OF GRANULATED SUGAR _7.10 OZ
- 1 LARGE EGG_ 1.7 OZ

BAKING PAN CONVERSION

- 9 -INCH ROUND CAKE PAN_ 12 CUPS
- 9 - INCH SPRINGFORM PAN _ 10 CUPS
- 10 - INCH TUBEPAN _ 16 CUPS

Printed by Amazon Italia Logistica S.r.l.
Torrazza Piemonte (TO), Italy

60572580R00054